It's easy to get lost in the cancer world

Let NCCN Guidelines for Patients® be your guide

- ✓ Step-by-step guides to the cancer care options likely to have the best results
- ✓ Based on treatment guidelines used by health care providers worldwide
- ✓ Designed to help you discuss cancer treatment with your doctors

About

National Comprehensive Cancer Network®

NCCN Guidelines for Patients® are developed by the National Comprehensive Cancer Network® (NCCN®)

NCCN

- An alliance of leading cancer centers across the United States devoted to patient care, research, and education

Cancer centers that are part of NCCN: NCCN.org/cancercenters

NCCN Clinical Practice Guidelines in Oncology (NCCN Guidelines®)

- Developed by doctors from NCCN cancer centers using the latest research and years of experience
- For providers of cancer care all over the world
- Expert recommendations for cancer screening, diagnosis, and treatment

Free online at NCCN.org/guidelines

NCCN Guidelines for Patients

- Present information from the NCCN Guidelines in an easy-to-learn format
- For people with cancer and those who support them
- Explain the cancer care options likely to have the best results

Free online at NCCN.org/patientguidelines

NATIONAL COMPREHENSIVE CANCER NETWORK FOUNDATION Guiding Treatment. Changing Lives.

and supported by funding from NCCN Foundation®

These NCCN Guidelines for Patients are based on the NCCN Guidelines® for Squamous Cell Skin Cancer (Version 2.2020, July 14, 2020).

NCCN Foundation seeks to support the millions of patients and their families affected by a cancer diagnosis by funding and distributing NCCN Guidelines for Patients. NCCN Foundation is also committed to advancing cancer treatment by funding the nation's promising doctors at the center of innovation in cancer research. For more details and the full library of patient and caregiver resources, visit NCCN.org/patients.

National Comprehensive Cancer Network (NCCN) / NCCN Foundation
3025 Chemical Road, Suite 100
Plymouth Meeting, PA 19462
215.690.0300

Endorsed by

Save Your Skin Foundation

Save Your Skin Foundation (SYSF) is a Canadian patient-led not-for-profit group dedicated to the fight against non-melanoma skin cancers, melanoma and ocular melanoma. By using and sharing the valuable and thorough NCCN Guidelines, SYSF is confident in their provision of solid patient support with accurate and current information on these cancers and related topics such as skin cancer treatment with immunotherapy. saveyourskin.ca

To make a gift or learn more, please visit NCCNFoundation.org/donate or e-mail PatientGuidelines@nccn.org.

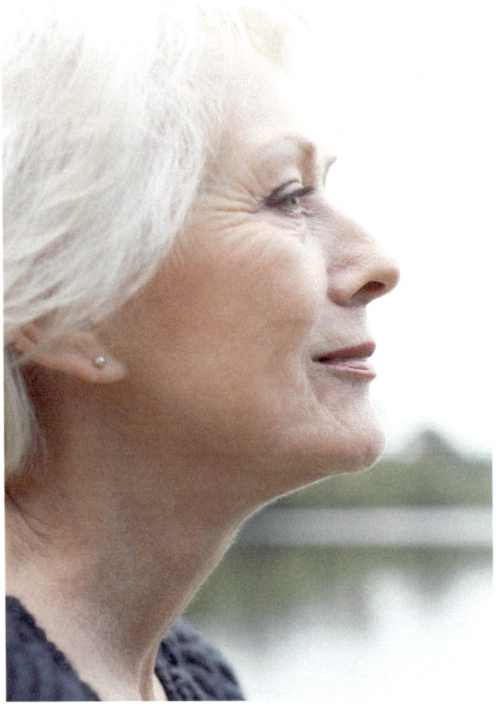
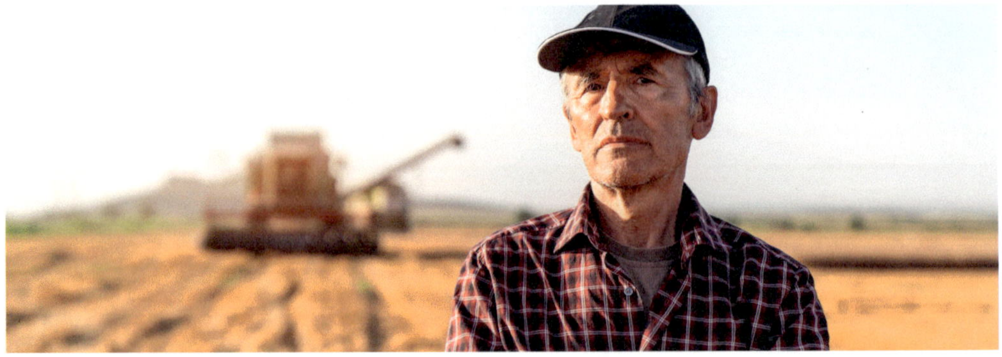
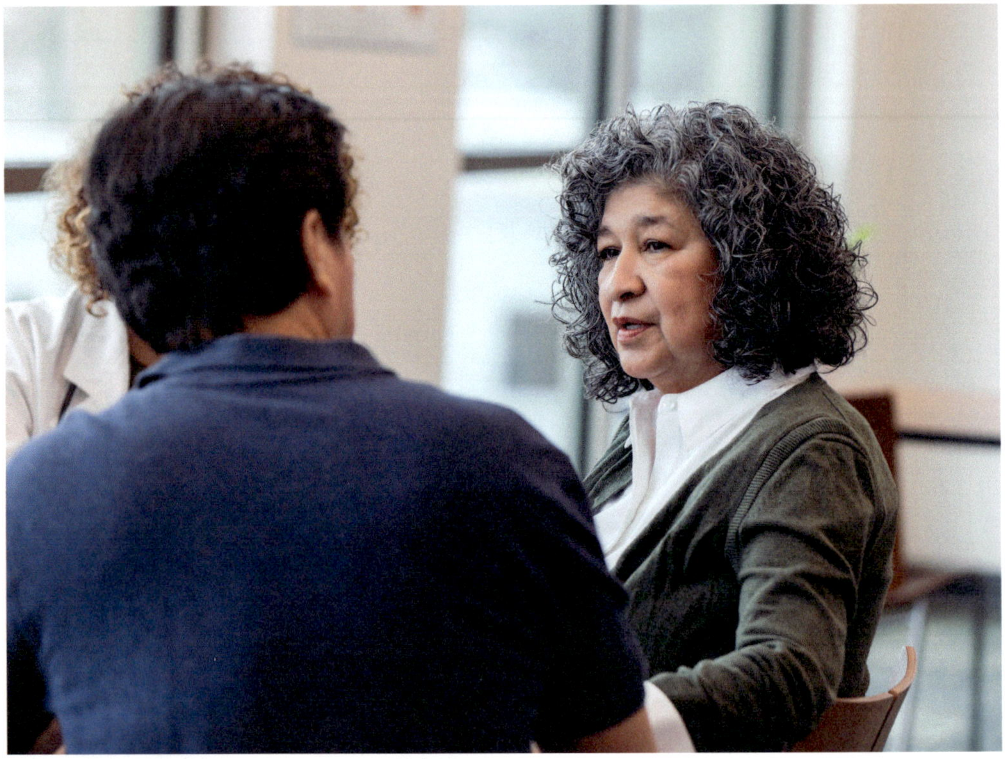
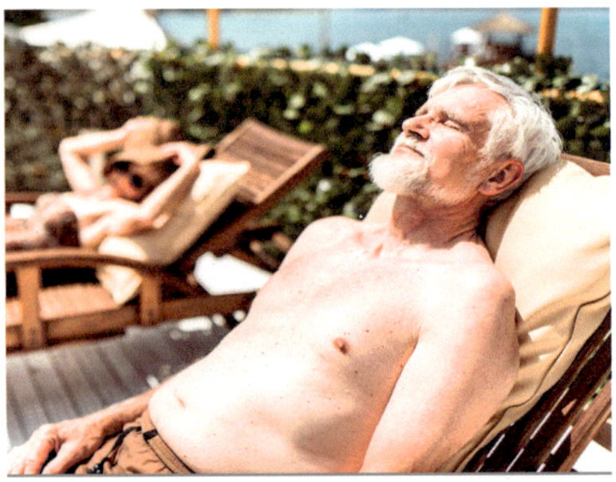
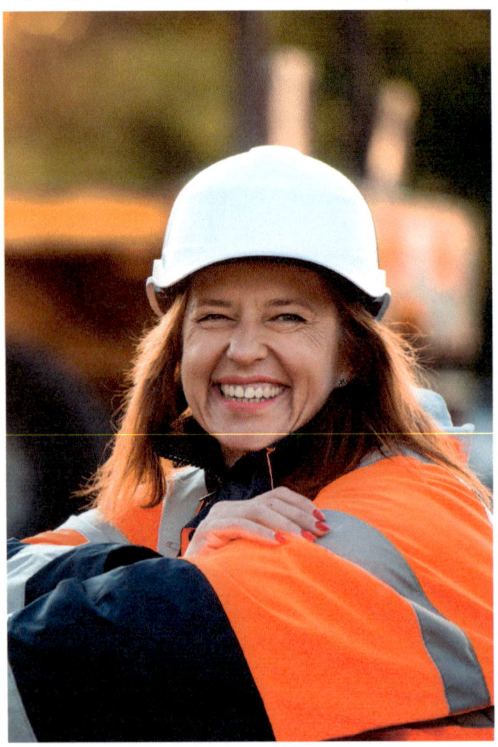
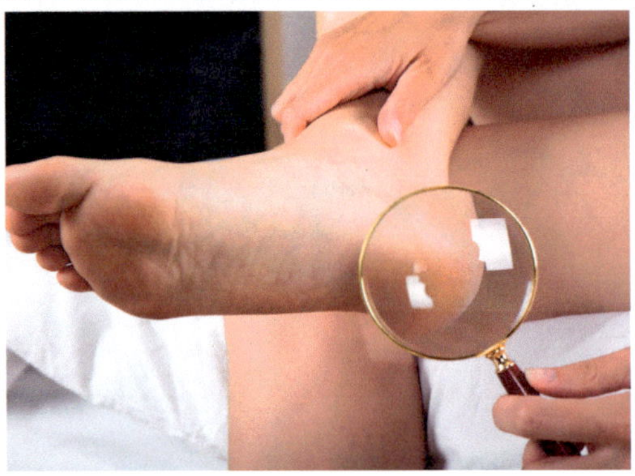
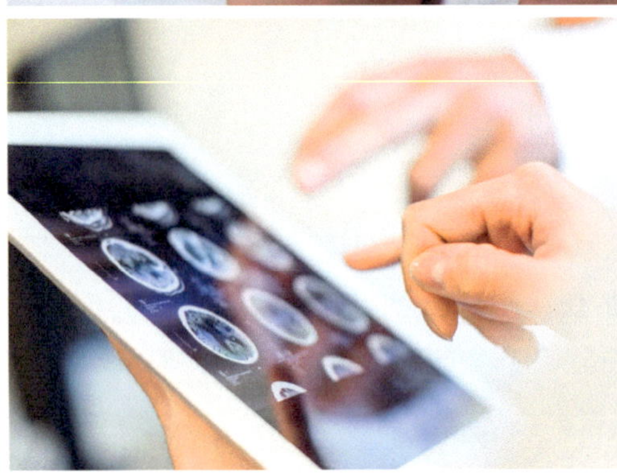
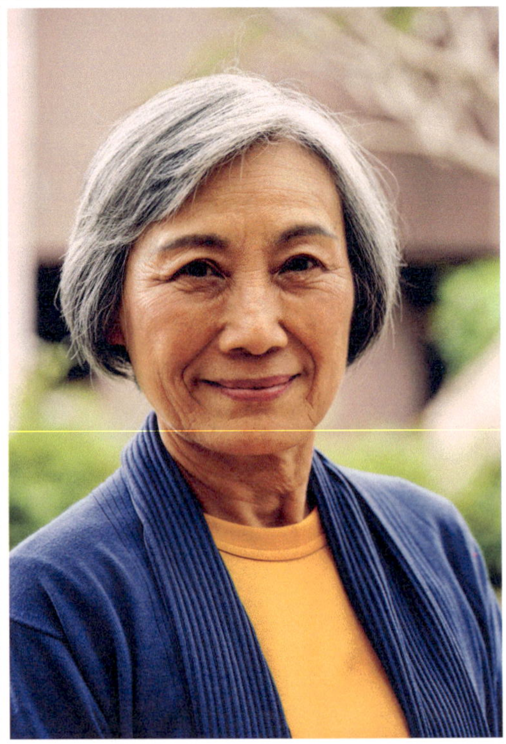

Contents

1
Squamous cell skin cancer basics

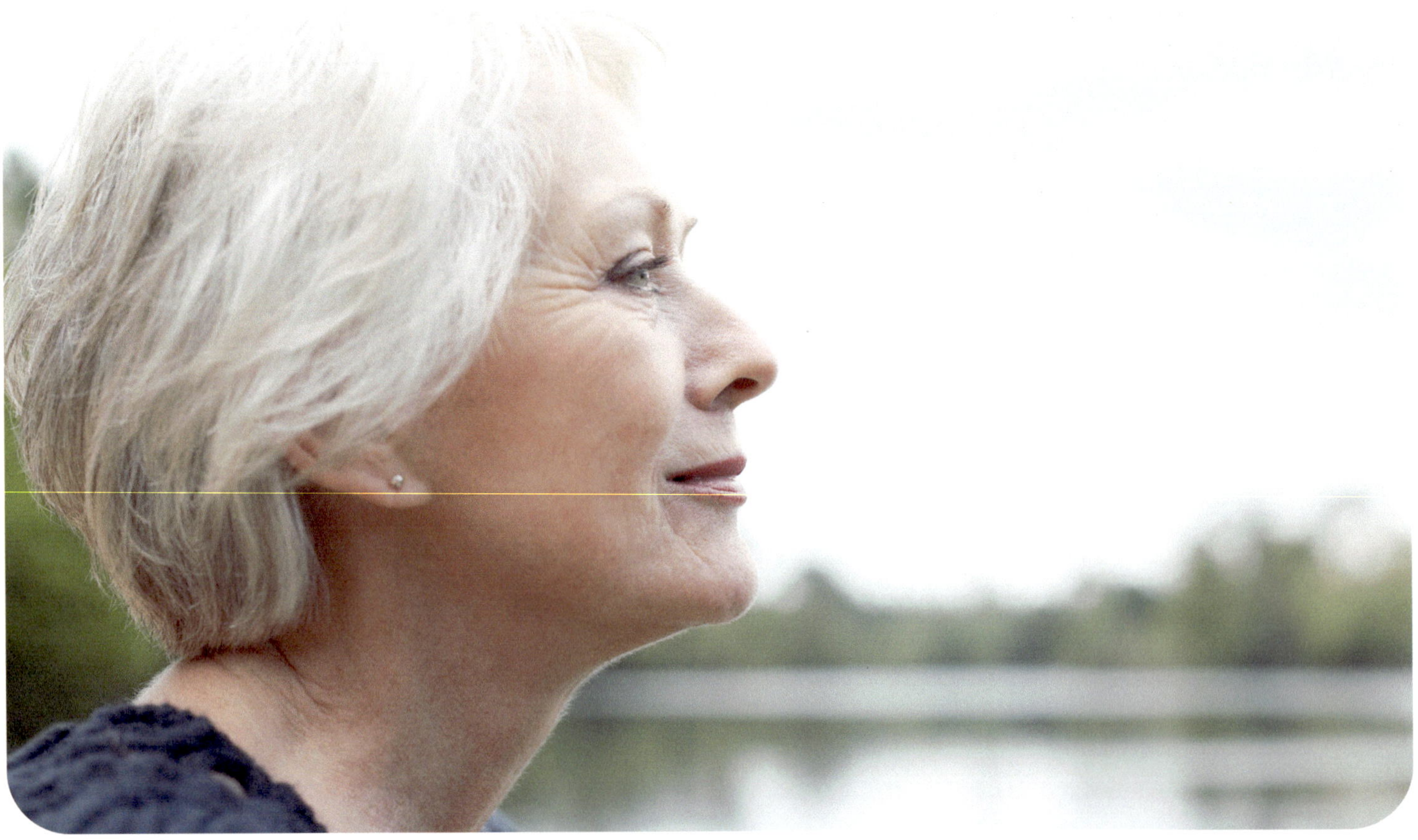

Cutaneous squamous cell carcinoma (cSCC) is the second most common type of skin cancer. It is highly treatable and can often be cured.

About

Squamous cell skin cancer is a very common skin cancer, especially in fair-skinned people. It is the second most common type of skin cancer, after basal cell carcinoma. The third type—melanoma—is rare but often more aggressive. Because they are so different from melanoma, basal cell and squamous cell skin cancers are referred to as non-melanoma skin cancers. This patient guide is about squamous cell skin cancer only. The terms "squamous cell skin cancer" and "cSCC" are used interchangeably throughout this guide.

There are three main layers of skin. Squamous cells and basal cells are found in the top-most layer (the epidermis). Squamous cells are also found in other areas of the body, such as the lungs, thyroid, and esophagus. Cancer that starts in a squamous cell is called a squamous cell carcinoma.

The dermis layer is below the epidermis. It contains hair follicles, nerves, sweat glands, oil glands, and blood vessels. Beneath the dermis is the "fatty" layer of skin (the subcutaneous tissue). This layer is best known for its many fat cells.

Layers and cell structure of skin

Squamous cells are found in the top layer of skin, called the epidermis.

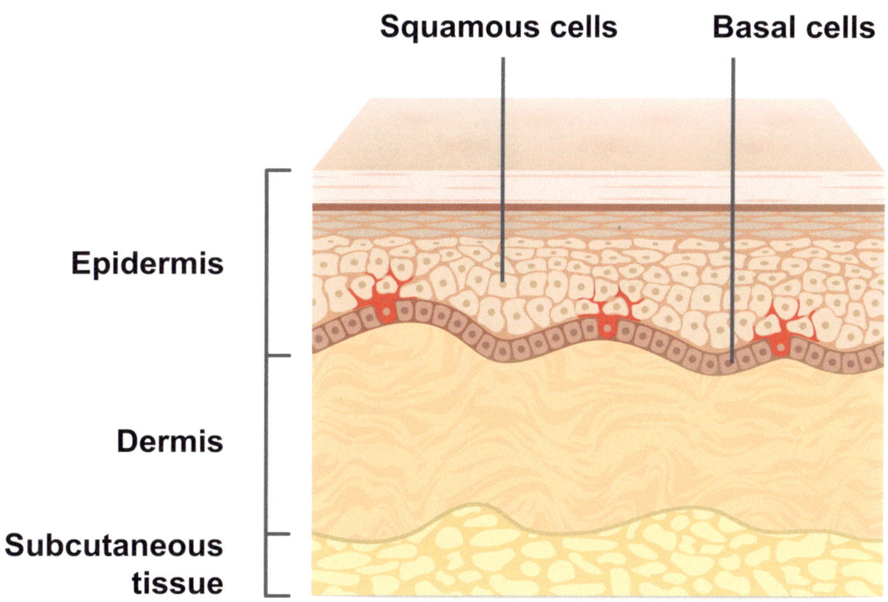

Who is at risk?

A risk factor is something that increases the chances of getting a particular disease. For example, smoking cigarettes is a risk factor for developing lung cancer. The major risk factors for squamous cell skin cancer are described next.

Sunlight

Most squamous cell skin cancers are caused by spending too much time in the sun over the course of many years, especially in people who sunburn easily. People with light skin, hair, and eyes who have been exposed to too much sun throughout their lives are at the highest risk for squamous cell skin cancer. People who work outdoors are also at higher risk. Because long-term sun exposure can lead to squamous cell skin cancer, it is more common in older people who have spent more years in the sun. Older people also may have weaker immune systems, which makes it easier for cancer to develop.

Indoor tanning

The use of tanning beds is a major risk factor for squamous cell skin cancer. All types of tanning (especially indoor tanning) increases the risk of getting any type of skin cancer.

Scars and chronic wounds

cSCC can form in scars or chronic (non-healing) wounds, such as ulcers (sores) and burns. This is known as Marjolin's ulcer. cSCC that starts in damaged, inflamed, or scarred skin is difficult to treat and more likely to come back after treatment.

Sun exposure

Most squamous cell skin cancers are caused by spending too much time in the sun over a long period of time.

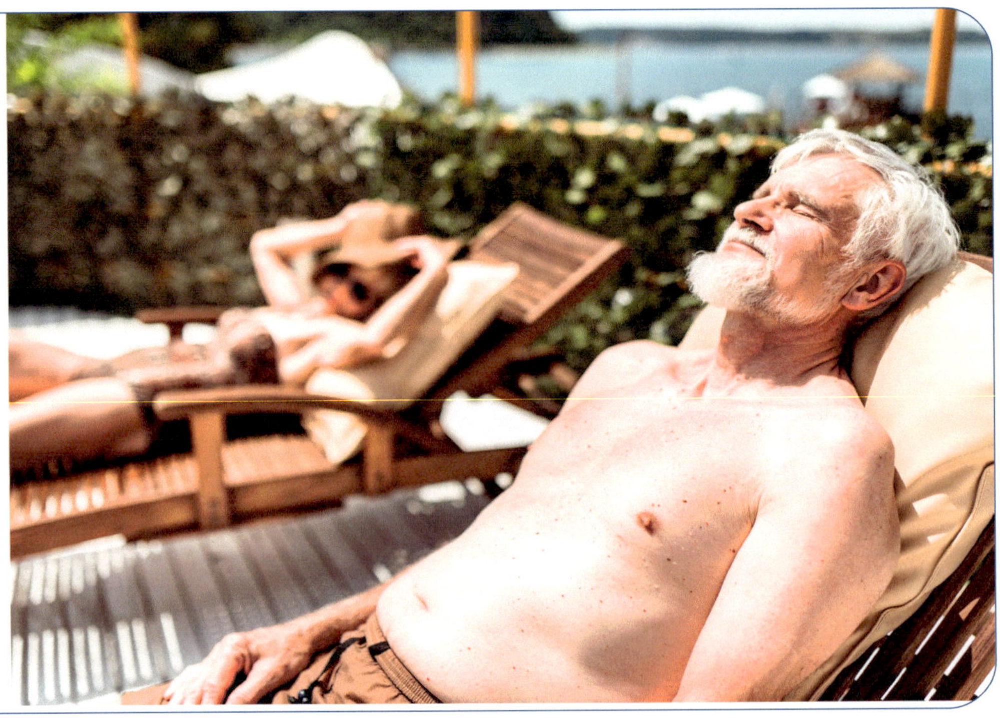

Actinic keratoses

An actinic keratosis is an area of rough skin caused by exposure to the sun over time. Actinic keratoses vary in appearance, and may be red, white, tan, or pink in color. They may appear as small scaly spots or stick out from the skin like bumps. Some may even look like warts. Having actinic keratoses means you are at higher risk of developing squamous cell skin cancer.

Bowen's disease

The earliest form of squamous cell skin cancer is called Bowen's disease. The cancer cells are only in the epidermis and have not invaded deeper layers of the skin. Bowen's disease is also known as cSCC in situ and stage 0 cSCC.

Genetic syndromes

Having certain genetic syndromes means you are at higher risk of getting squamous cell skin cancer. One such syndrome is albinism (lack of color in the hair, skin, and eyes). Another is xeroderma pigmentosum, in which the body is not able to repair damage to deoxyribonucleic acid (DNA) caused by sunlight. Skin cells with a lot of DNA damage can eventually become skin cancers.

Weakened immune system

Having a weakened immune system can put you at risk of squamous cell skin cancer. An example of this is organ transplantation. If you received an organ from another person, you likely take drugs to stop your body from attacking the donated organ. These drugs, called immunosuppressants, also reduce the

Actinic keratosis on hand

An actinic keratosis is an area of rough skin caused by being in the sun over time.

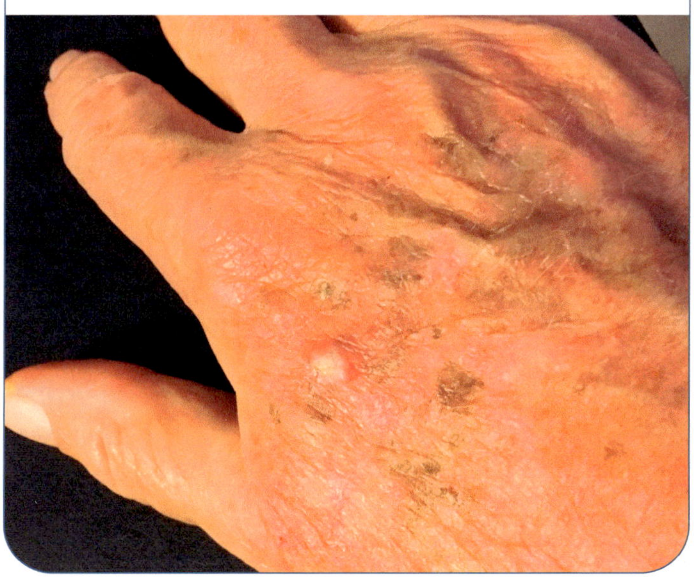

Actinic keratosis on top of head

Actinic keratoses can vary in appearance and may be red, white, tan, or pink in color.

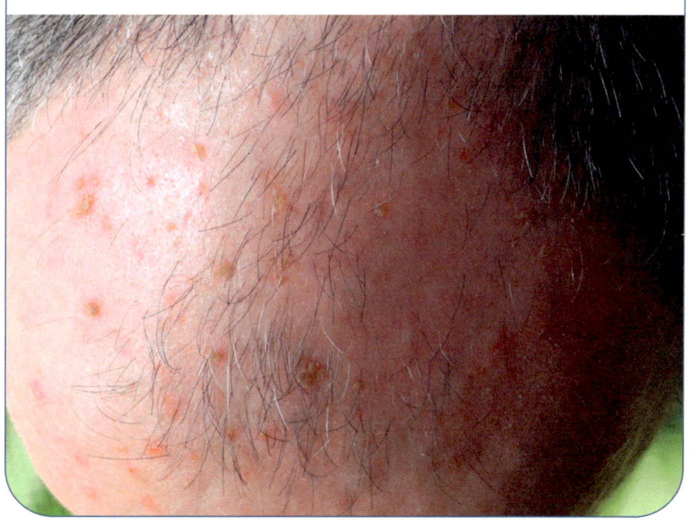

body's ability to fight infection and disease. Your immune system also may not work well because of other medical conditions, such as lymphoma, chronic lymphocytic leukemia, and human immunodeficiency virus (HIV). Any of these increases the risk of getting squamous cell skin cancer.

Diagnosis

An area of abnormal skin is called a lesion. If a lesion suspicious for skin cancer is found, testing may include:

- A close examination of the lesion(s)
- A head-to-toe skin exam to look for other lesions
- A lymph node exam
- A full health history
- A skin biopsy (removal and testing of a sample of the lesion)
- Imaging test (if there is suspicion that the cancer has grown deep into the skin or has spread to lymph nodes or other parts of the body)

Cancer cells can travel through blood and lymph to form tumors in other parts of the body. If your lymph nodes feel larger than they should or look suspicious on imaging tests, cancer may have spread to the lymph nodes. To find out, your doctor will use a needle to take a sample from the lymph node for testing (a lymph node biopsy). Squamous cell skin cancer that has not spread to nearby lymph nodes is referred to as "local". See page 20 for information on local cSCC. If cancer is found in the lymph node, it is called "regional" squamous cell skin cancer. See page 25 for information on regional cSCC.

SNAPSHOT

Cutaneous squamous cell carcinoma (cSCC)

- A very common type of skin cancer, especially in light-skinned people
- More commonly found in areas of the body exposed to sun, especially the head and neck
- Over 95% of people can be cured by completely removing the cSCC
- Rarely spreads to distant areas of the body
- Can spread in the area where it forms, causing severe damage and, in rare cases, death

Review

- Squamous cell skin cancer is the second most common type of skin cancer. It is highly treatable and can often be cured.
- Squamous cell skin cancer is most commonly caused by getting sunburns or spending too much time in the sun over many years.
- An actinic keratosis is an area of scaly or rough skin that has a higher chance of becoming squamous cell skin cancer.
- Bowen's disease is the earliest form of squamous cell skin cancer. The cancer cells have not invaded deeper layers of the skin.
- You may be more likely to get squamous cell skin cancer if you have a weakened immune system, certain genetic syndromes, or actinic keratoses.
- Squamous cell skin cancer can form in old wounds, burns, or scars. This is called Marjolin's ulcer and it tends to be harder to treat.

2
Overview of treatments

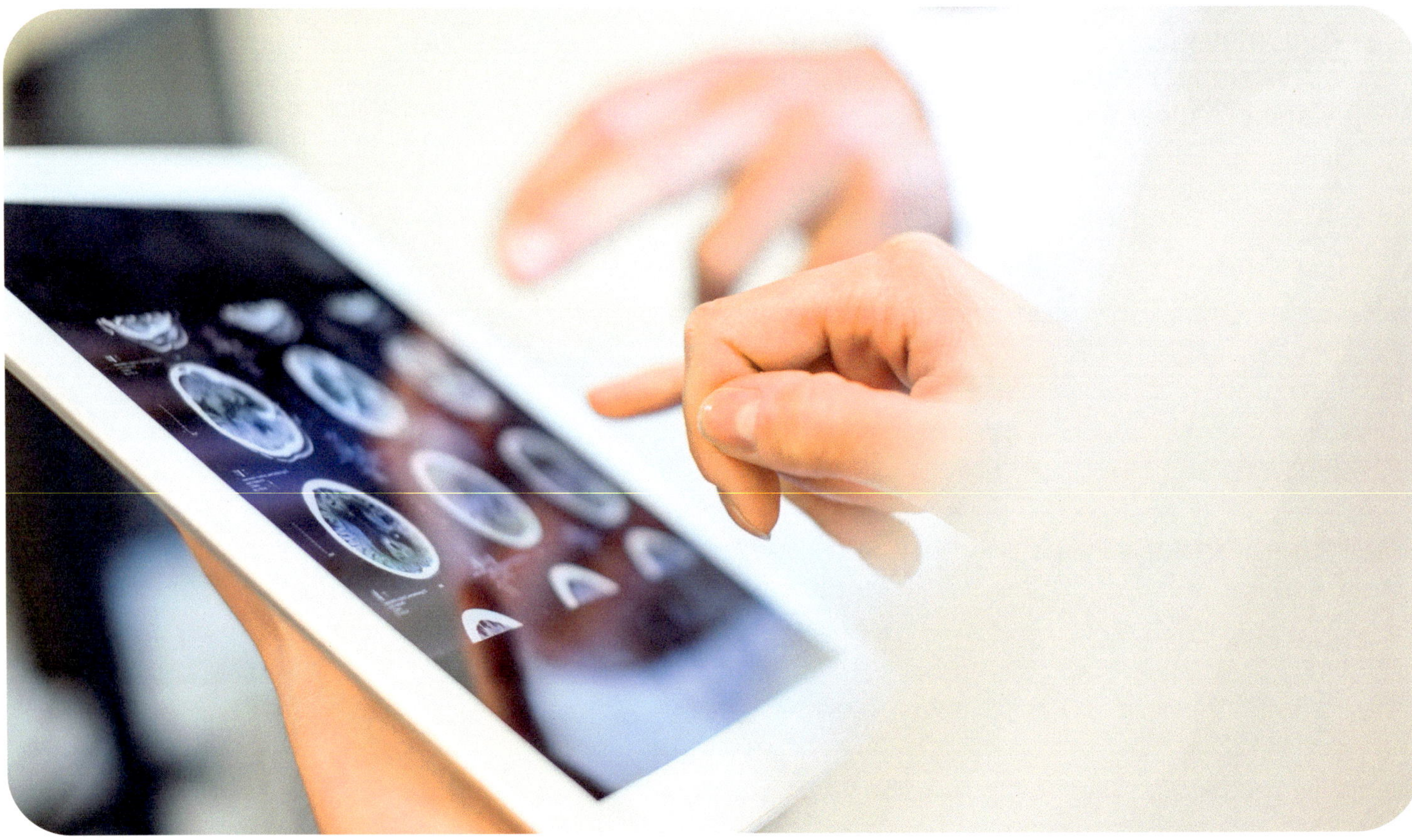

This chapter describes the treatments for squamous cell skin cancer. The best treatment for you will depend on the extent of the cancer, whether surgery is a suitable option, and your personal preferences.

Superficial treatments

Treatments that affect only the top layer of the skin are called superficial treatments. Patients with the earliest form of squamous cell skin cancer (Bowen's disease) tend to also have have actinic keratoses (pre-cancerous lesions) in the same general area. While surgery is preferred to treat more advanced cSCC, superficial treatments are additional options often used to treat Bowen's disease and actinic keratoses.

Photodynamic therapy

In photodynamic therapy (PDT), a light-sensitive drug is applied to the area. When exposed to light (either red or blue light in the doctor's office, or shaded outdoor light), the drug becomes active and kills cancer cells. Common side effects of PDT include itching or burning when the liquid is applied, pain during the red or blue light exposure, and itching and redness for a few days after treatment.

Cryotherapy

Cryotherapy (also called cryosurgery) freezes and destroys cancerous cells using a very cold liquid or tool. Liquid nitrogen is frequently used. Cryotherapy causes a burning sensation during treatment and then a blister and scab forms and heals over 2 to 3 weeks. Skin darkening or lightening can occur upon healing.

Topical therapies

Imiquimod (Aldara®) and 5-fluorouracil (also known as 5-FU) are prescription chemotherapy creams used to treat Bowen's disease and

Photodynamic therapy

A drug applied to the skin becomes active and kills cancer cells when exposed to light.

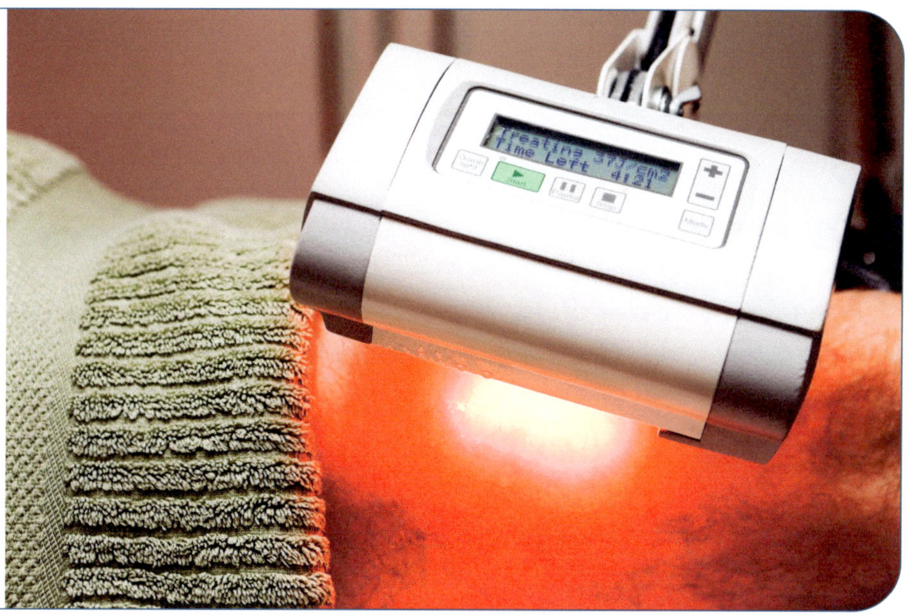

actinic keratoses. Imiquimod belongs to a group of drugs known as immune response modifiers. This cream is thought to help fight abnormal skin growths by activating the immune system to damage abnormal skin cells.

5-fluorouracil (Carac®, Efudex®, Fluoroplex®) is a type of topical chemotherapy. It is applied directly to the skin, unlike traditional chemotherapy which is put into the bloodstream. For the treatment of actinic keratosis, 5-fluorouracil is often used with another topical therapy called calcipotriene (Sorilux™, Dovonex®). Calcipotriene is a form of vitamin D that activates the skin's immune system.

Ingenol mebutate (Picato®) is another topical therapy used to treat actinic keratosis. This prescription gel is applied directly to the skin once daily for 2 to 3 days.

Thickening of the outer layer of skin is known as hyperkeratosis. For hyperkeratotic (thick and rough) actinic keratoses, one or more of the following may be used before treatment with the therapies described above. The goal is to soften and break down the thick top layer before treatment.

- Topical tazarotene (a retinoid product related to vitamin A)
- Curettage (scraping away skin with a spoon-shaped tool)
- Topical keratolytics (topical urea, lactic acid, or salicylic acid)

Other therapies that are sometimes used for actinic keratoses include topical diclofenac, chemical peels (trichloroacetic acid), and resurfacing techniques such as laser or dermabrasion.

Topical therapies for squamous cell skin cancer can cause burning, redness, itching, and pain in the treated area. Sun-damaged skin may need to be re-treated with topical therapies from time to time.

Cryotherapy

Cryotherapy freezes and destroys cancer cells using a very cold liquid or tool.

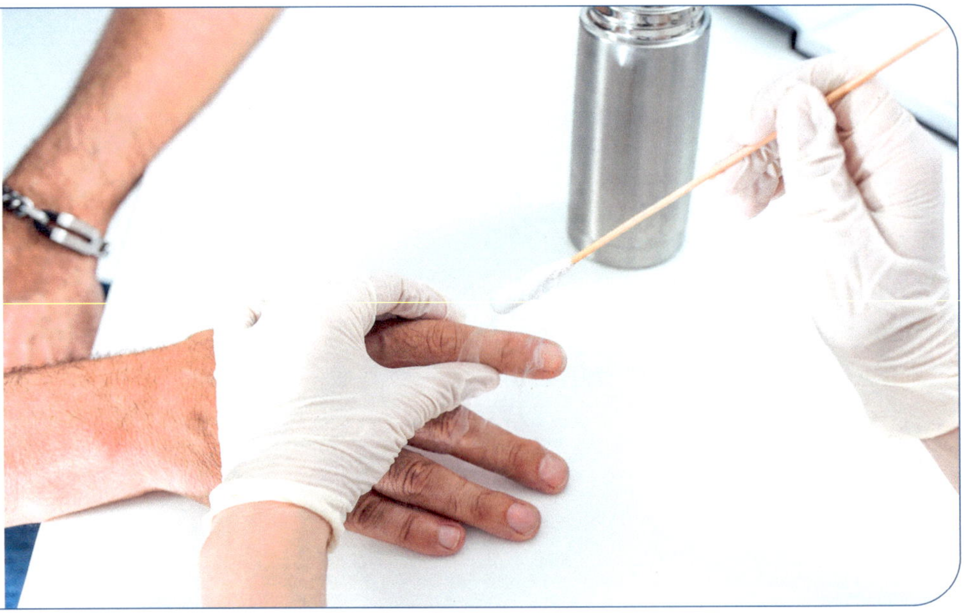

Surgery

Curettage and electrodesiccation (C&E)

C&E is done in a medical office with local numbing to the area. In this method, the visible tumor is first scraped off using a thin tool with a sharp loop or spoon at the end. Next, an electric needle is used to cauterize (burn) the base of the wound. This usually kills any remaining cancer cells and helps stop bleeding. This two-step system of scraping then burning may be done up to three times in the same session. Curettage and electrodesiccation is a recommended treatment option for low-risk cSCC that has not spread to lymph nodes. If the tumor ends up being deeper than expected during C&E, a standard surgical excision may be needed to remove deep areas of cancerous tissue.

Mohs surgery

Mohs surgery can be done in a medical office or surgical suite. Most patients remain awake during the procedure. After the area is numbed, the visible tumor is first removed using a scalpel. Next, a thin layer of surrounding tissue is removed from under and around the wound. The edges and underside of this tissue are evaluated by the Mohs surgeon using a microscope while you wait. If cancer cells are seen by the surgeon, another thin layer of tissue is removed only from the area of the wound where the cancer was seen. When a removed layer shows no cancer cells at its edges, the procedure is over. The wound can be closed in many ways. Some may heal better without stitches. Other wounds may need skin grafts or other types of surgery to heal well and minimize scars. This may be done the same day or a few days after the Mohs procedure.

Mohs surgery is a recommended treatment option for high-risk cSCC that has not spread to lymph nodes. It is often used for cSCC on the head, face, hands, feet, shins, and genital areas because it can remove the cancer while sparing as much normal tissue as possible. Mohs surgery may also be used after standard surgical excision (described next) in both high-

Mohs surgery

This procedure allows the surgeon to know right away whether all cancer was removed.

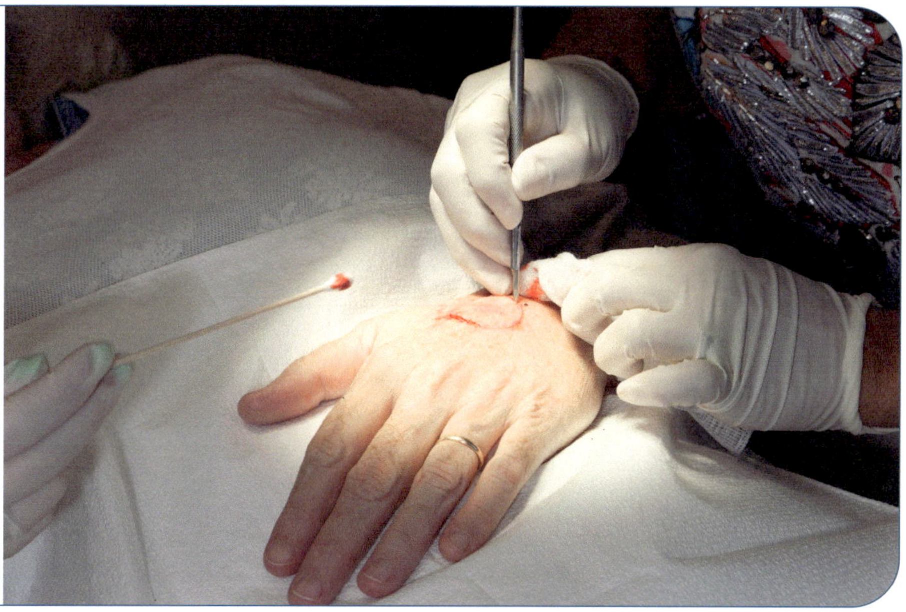

and low-risk patients, if the excision did not remove all of the cancer.

Resection with CCPDMA

Another option is excision with complete circumferential peripheral and deep margin assessment (CCPDMA). Like Mohs surgery, this procedure allows for complete testing of the edges of removed tissue.

Standard surgical excision

A standard surgical excision (removal) can be done in a medical office while you are awake. After the area is numbed, the doctor removes the tumor and an area of normal tissue surrounding it with a scalpel blade. The edges of the removed tissue are called the surgical margin. A wider margin (area of normal tissue around the lesion) is removed for high-risk cSCC. The tissue is then sent for testing. A pathologist examines thin samples of the tissue under a microscope to see if there are cancer cells at the margin. If there are, it is called a positive margin and more treatment is needed. Next treatments you have may include Mohs surgery (or resection with CCPDMA) or another surgical excision. If you cannot have more surgery, radiation therapy is an option. Standard surgical excision is almost always an option for treating squamous cell skin cancer.

Radiation therapy

Radiation therapy uses photons (high-energy x-rays), electrons, or protons (charged particles) to kill cancer cells. There are two general types of radiation therapy that can be used to treat cSCC: external beam radiation therapy (EBRT) and brachytherapy. In EBRT, a beam of radiation is directed at the tumor from a machine. In brachytherapy, a radiation source is placed close to or in direct contact with the tumor for a short period of time. The two most common types of external beam radiation for cSCC are electrons and photons. Electrons are used to treat superficial tumors. Photons are used to treat deeper, more invasive tumors.

Mohs surgery

Mohs surgery is one of the recommended treatment options for high-risk cSCC that has not spread to lymph nodes.

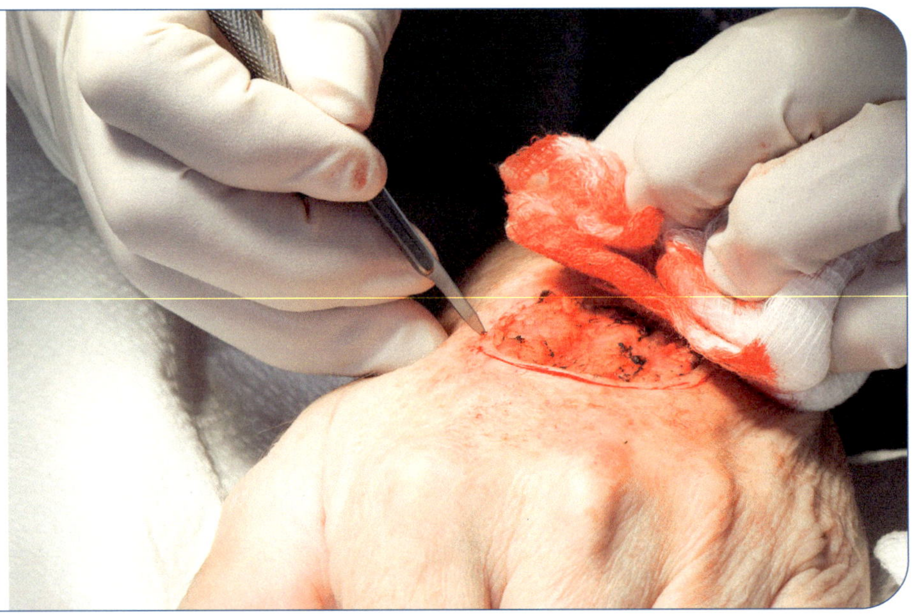

Radiation therapy is an option for people who cannot or choose not to have surgery. The cure rate is generally lower compared to surgery. However, radiation therapy can be very effective for small tumors. Radiation is sometimes used after surgery to kill any remaining cancer cells, or to help prevent recurrence for patients with high-risk tumors.

Radiation therapy usually involves 5 daily brief treatments per week over 3 to 7 weeks. The most common short-term side effects of radiation are redness of the skin, itching, mild discomfort, and mild to moderate fatigue. These side effects are worst at the end of the radiation course and take several weeks to go away.

Potential long-term side effects of radiation include hardening of the skin and soft tissue in the treatment area, mild change in skin color (usually lightening), and spider veins. More serious potential long-term side effects include non-healing ulcers and cataracts (for cSCC in the eye area). Rarely, patients treated with radiation can develop a second skin cancer in the treated area. This is more common in young patients many years (decades) later.

Radiation therapy should not be used in people with certain conditions that put them at higher risk of skin cancer caused by radiation, such as basal cell nevus syndrome or xeroderma pigmentosum. It may also not be appropriate for some people with connective tissue diseases, such as lupus or scleroderma.

The same area generally should not be treated with radiation more than once. When cSCC grows in a radiated area, it usually needs to be removed with surgery. However, the area often doesn't heal as well because the tissues were weakened by the radiation. This is especially true for cSCC on the scalp.

Systemic therapy

Systemic therapy is treatment with medicine(s) that travel in the bloodstream to reach cells throughout the body. Systemic therapies can impact both cancer cells and normal cells, resulting in side effects. Chemotherapy, targeted therapy, and immunotherapy are systemic therapies.

They are given intravenously (through the veins) or taken by mouth as a pill. Systemic therapy is not used often to treat squamous cell skin cancer. It may be an option if surgery and radiation therapy are not possible, or were not successful. It may also be used in combination with radiation therapy to treat cSCC that cannot be removed using surgery.

Chemotherapy

Some chemotherapy medicines contain the metal platinum. Cisplatin and carboplatin are platinum chemotherapies used to treat squamous cell skin cancer and other cancers. They may be given in combination with other chemotherapy drugs.

Targeted therapy

Targeted therapies are medicines that can target and attack specific types of receptors on cancer cells. The targeted therapies used to treat squamous cell skin cancer are known as epidermal growth factor receptor (EGFR) inhibitors. EGFR is a protein found on the surface of cells that causes them to divide. Inhibiting (blocking) EGFR may keep cancer cells from growing. Cetuximab (Erbitux®) is an EGFR inhibitor used to treat cSCC and other cancers.

Immunotherapy

Immunotherapy stimulates the activity of the immune system, which can improve the body's ability to find and destroy cancer cells. Immunotherapies used to treat cSCC and other cancers are known as PD-1 inhibitors. PD-1 inhibitors are a type of immune checkpoint inhibitor. Cemiplimab (Libtayo®) and pembrolizumab (Keytruda®) are PD-1 inhibitors used to treat squamous cell skin cancer and other cancers.

Side effects of systemic therapy

The side effects of systemic therapy vary greatly depending on the medicine(s) used. Side effects may include:

- Tiredness (fatigue)
- Nausea and vomiting
- Lung and breathing problems (cough, shortness of breath, chest pain)
- Damage to major organs including the liver and kidneys
- Hair loss
- Mouth sores
- Body aches
- Rash and other skin problems
- Loss of appetite
- Diarrhea
- Constipation
- Low blood cell counts
- High blood pressure
- Abnormal bleeding
- Side effects of immunotherapy known as immune-related adverse events (irAEs)

Not all side effects are discussed here. If systemic therapy is planned, ask you care team for a complete list. While most side effects start when treatment starts and stop when it is over, some can occur years later. Long-term side effects of systemic therapy can include other cancers, heart disease, and infertility.

For more information on side effects of immune checkpoint inhibitors, see *the NCCN Guidelines for Patients Immunotherapy Side Effects: Immune Checkpoint Inhibitors* at NCCN.org/patientguidelines.

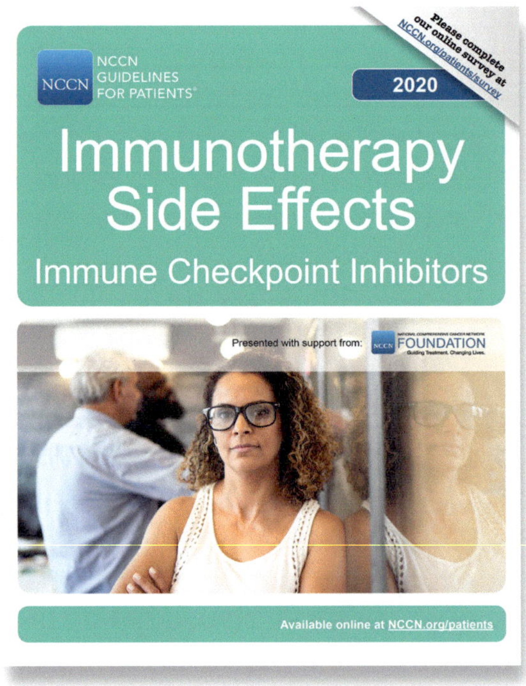

Clinical trials

New tests and treatments are not offered to the public as they are made. They first need to be studied. A clinical trial is a type of research that studies how safe and helpful tests and treatments are. When found to be safe and helpful, they may become tomorrow's standard of care. Because of clinical trials, the tests and treatments in this book are now widely used to help people with cancer.

Joining a clinical trial can have both benefits and risks. You will need to weigh the pros and cons and decide what is right for you.

To join a clinical trial, you must meet the conditions of the study, or eligibility criteria. Patients in a clinical trial are often alike in terms of their cancer and general health. This is to know that any progress is because of the treatment and not because of differences between patients.

To join you will need to discuss with your provider and review and sign a paper called an informed consent. This form describes the study in detail. The study's risks and benefits should be described and may include others than those described above.

Ask your treatment team if there is a clinical trial that you can join. There may be clinical trials at the medical center where you are getting treatment or at other treatment centers nearby. You can also find clinical trials through the websites listed in the last chapter of this book.

Review

- Photodynamic therapy, cryotherapy, and topical therapy are treatment options for Bowen's disease and actinic keratoses (pre-cancerous lesions).
- Types of surgery for squamous cell skin cancer include curettage and electrodesiccation, Mohs surgery, and standard surgical excision.
- Radiation therapy is a treatment option for people who cannot or choose not to have surgery. For the treatment of some squamous cell skin cancers, it is used after surgery to kill remaining cancer cells.
- Systemic therapy (eg, chemotherapy, targeted therapy, immunotherapy) is not used often for cSCC, except when it has spread elsewhere in the body. It may be an option if surgery and radiation therapy are not possible, or were not successful.

3 Treatment guide: Local cSCC

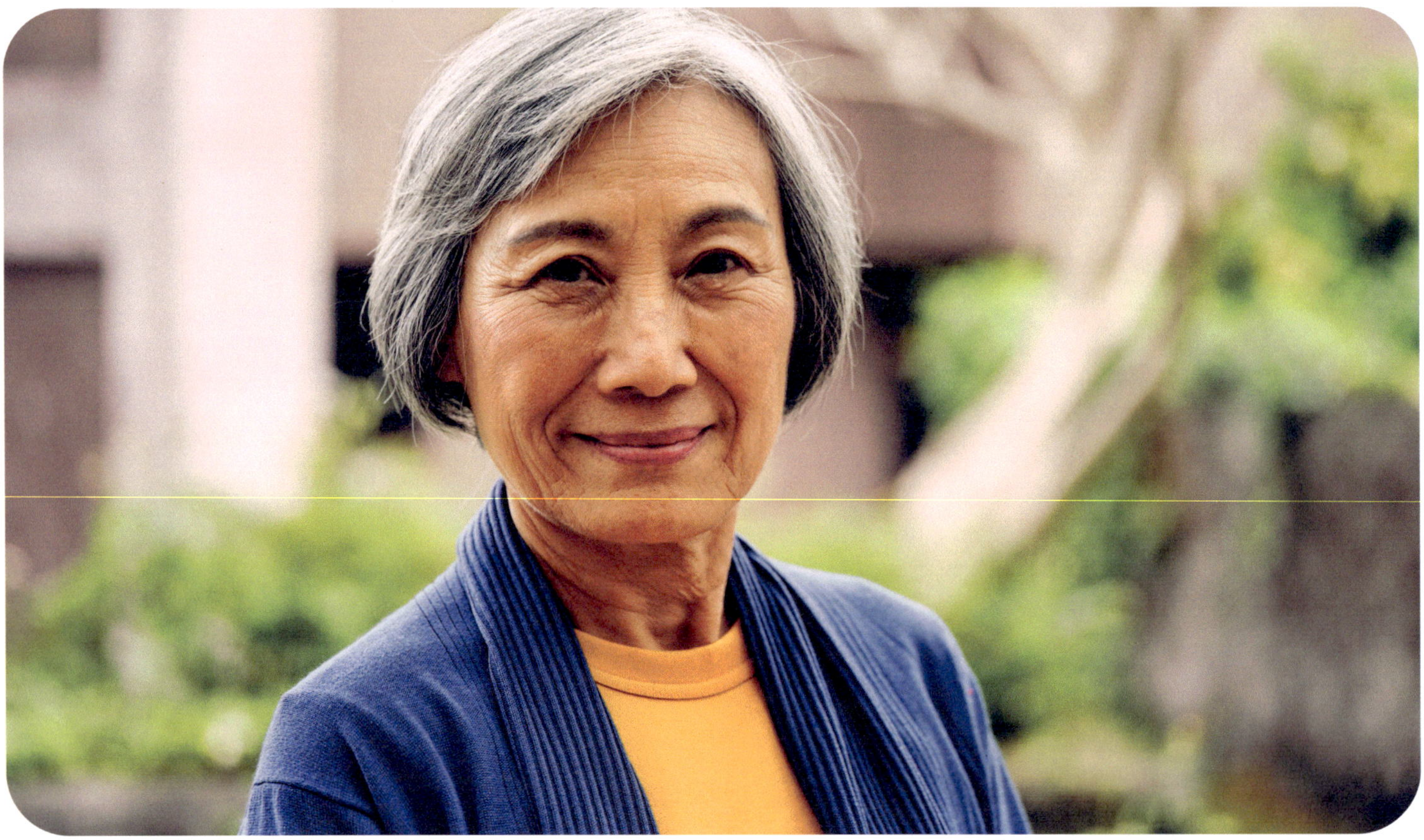

Squamous cell skin cancer that has not spread to nearby lymph nodes is known as "local". Local disease is usually treated with surgery. The goal of treatment is to remove all of the cancer with as little damage to the surrounding skin as possible.

Risk assessment

Based on the features of the cancer, some people will be at higher risk of the cancer returning after treatment and spreading to distant areas (metastasis). After squamous cell skin cancer is confirmed, your doctor will consider several features of the cancer to determine if it is a low- or high-risk skin cancer. This is important to know because high-risk disease is treated differently than low-risk disease.

The following factors are used to determine your risk level. If your cancer has any of the risk factors described below, it is a high-risk squamous cell carcinoma.

Location and size

Squamous cell skin cancer on the head or neck is more likely to return after treatment than tumors on the trunk, arms, or legs. The following tumors are considered high risk because of their location and size:

- Tumors on the trunk, arms, or legs that are 20 mm (about the size of a nickel) or larger
- Tumors on the cheeks, forehead, scalp, neck, or shins that are 10 mm (about the size of a pea) or larger
- Any tumor on the hands, feet, sex organs, or the "mask area" of the face (includes the eyelids, eyebrows, nose, lips, chin, and temples)

Tumor return after treatment

Any tumor that has returned after treatment is considered a high-risk squamous cell skin cancer.

Weakened immune system

People with a weakened immune system are at increased risk of getting cSCC. They are also at higher risk of the cancer returning after treatment and spreading to distant sites. Examples of conditions that weaken the immune system include:

- Long-term corticosteroid use
- Human immunodeficiency virus (HIV)
- Having received an organ transplant

Tumor formed in damaged skin

If squamous cell skin cancer starts in an area that was previously treated with radiation therapy, it is considered a high-risk cancer. This is also the case if the cancer starts in a wound, a scar, or an area of damaged or inflamed skin.

Nerve damage

If the tumor has grown into a nerve or group of nerves, usually seen under the microscope, it is a high-risk cancer. This is known as perineural invasion. Signs that the cancer may have invaded nerves include pain, burning, stinging, loss of feeling, burning or pricking sensation, loss of movement, double vision, and blurred vision.

Tumor grade

The tumor grade is a rating of how fast your doctors expect the cancer to grow and spread. It is based on how different the tumor cells look compared to normal cells under a microscope. The more different they look, the higher the risk of spreading.

Tumor type

To diagnose squamous cell skin cancer, you likely had a small sample of tissue removed for testing (a skin biopsy). That tissue sample was then analyzed by a pathologist in order to determine the specific type (and sub-type) of cancer. There are certain rare subtypes of squamous cell skin cancer that are more likely to return after treatment.

Connective tissue in the tumor

Some tumors form fibrous or connective tissue, which is a sign of a high-risk cancer.

How deep the tumor has grown into the skin

The deeper the tumor has invaded into the skin, the higher the risk of the cancer returning after treatment or spreading to distant sites.

Cancer cells in lymph or blood vessels

If there are cancer cells in the blood vessels or lymph vessels outside of the main tumor, it means that the cancer is more likely to spread to nearby lymph nodes and other parts of the body. This is known as lymphovascular invasion.

Low-risk local cSCC

Surgery is the preferred treatment for low-risk cSCC that has not spread to lymph nodes. The options for surgery include:

- Curettage and electrodesiccation (C&E)
- Standard surgical excision

See pages 15 and 16 for detailed descriptions of these treatments. If you are not a candidate for surgery, treatment with radiation therapy is recommended if you can have it.

Curettage and electrodesiccation

C&E is a recommended treatment option for low-risk, local cSCC in areas without significant hair growth. If the tumor ends up being deeper than expected during the procedure, a standard surgical excision may be needed to remove deep areas of cancerous tissue.

Standard surgical excision

Standard surgical excision is a recommended treatment option for low-risk, local cSCC. If testing after surgery finds cancer cells in the surrounding tissue removed with the tumor, more treatment is needed. Treatment options include:

- Mohs surgery or resection with CCPDMA
- Another surgical excision
- Radiation therapy (if more surgery cannot be done)

➲ See *When treatment is over* on page 29 for information on monitoring and follow-up care.

High-risk local cSCC

Surgery is the preferred treatment for high-risk cSCC that has not spread to lymph nodes. The options for surgery include:

- Mohs surgery or resection with CCPDMA
- Standard surgical excision

If you are not a candidate for surgery, see *If surgery is not an option* on the next page.

Mohs surgery or resection with CCPDMA

Mohs surgery and resection with CCPDMA are recommended treatment options for high-risk local cSCC.

If Mohs surgery (or resection with CCPDMA) is successful at removing the cancer but other concerning features are noted during surgery, a discussion with different cancer physicians is recommended to determine next steps. Treatment with radiation therapy will be considered.

If Mohs surgery (or resection with CCPDMA) does not remove all of the cancer, a discussion between different cancer physicians is recommended to consider your treatment options. If another surgery can be performed, this is often tried first. Otherwise, radiation therapy is recommended. In some cases, systemic therapy is used in addition to radiation. Platinum-based chemotherapy is a recommended option for use with radiation if you can have it. Enrolling in a clinical trial for systemic therapy is also an option. A clinical trial could involve treatment with chemotherapy, targeted therapy, or immunotherapy.

If radiation therapy is not expected to kill the cancer completely or may damage critical healthy organs, systemic therapy alone is recommended. If you are eligible, immunotherapy with an immune checkpoint inhibitor is a recommended treatment option. Enrolling in a clinical trial for systemic therapy is also an option.

Standard surgical excision

Standard surgical excision is a recommended treatment option for high-risk local cSCC. A wider margin (area of normal tissue around the lesion) is removed for high-risk cSCC.

If standard surgical excision is successful at removing the cancer but other concerning features are noted during surgery, a discussion with different cancer physicians is recommended to determine next steps. Treatment with radiation therapy will be considered.

If testing after surgery finds cancer in the margin, more treatment is needed. If Mohs surgery (or resection with CCPDMA) is possible, it is usually tried first. Otherwise, another standard surgical excision is typically performed.

If cancer still remains and more surgery is not possible, a discussion between different cancer physicians to consider next steps is recommended. Treatment may include radiation therapy with or without systemic therapy. If systemic therapy is planned, platinum-based chemotherapy is a recommended option for use with radiation. Enrolling in a clinical trial for systemic therapy is also an option. A clinical trial could involve treatment with chemotherapy, targeted therapy, or immunotherapy.

If radiation therapy is not expected to kill the cancer completely or may damage critical healthy organs, systemic therapy alone is recommended. Immunotherapy with an immune checkpoint inhibitor is a recommended treatment option if you are eligible. Enrolling in a clinical trial for systemic therapy is also an option.

If surgery is not an option

If you are not a candidate for surgery, radiation therapy is typically used instead. Systemic therapy may be given in addition to radiation. If systemic therapy is planned, platinum-based chemotherapy is a recommended option for use with radiation. Enrolling in a clinical trial for systemic therapy is also an option. A clinical trial could involve treatment with chemotherapy, targeted therapy, or immunotherapy.

If radiation therapy is not expected to kill the cancer completely or may damage critical healthy organs, systemic therapy alone is recommended. If you are eligible, immunotherapy with an immune checkpoint inhibitor is a recommended treatment option. Enrolling in a clinical trial for systemic therapy is also an option.

➲ See *When treatment is over* on page 29 for information on monitoring and follow-up care.

Review

- Squamous cell skin cancer that has not spread to nearby lymph nodes is known as "local".
- Local cSCC is most often treated with surgery.
- Key features of the cancer will be considered to determine if it is a low- or high-risk cSCC. This is called a risk assessment.
- Recommended types of surgery for local, low-risk cSCC include curettage and electrodesiccation (C&E) and standard surgical excision.
- For low-risk cSCC in non-surgical candidates, treatment with radiation therapy is an option.
- Recommended types of surgery for local, high-risk cSCC include Mohs surgery, resection with CCPDMA, and standard surgical excision.
- For high-risk cSCC in non-surgical candidates, treatment with radiation therapy and/or systemic therapy is an option.

4 Treatment guide: cSCC in lymph nodes

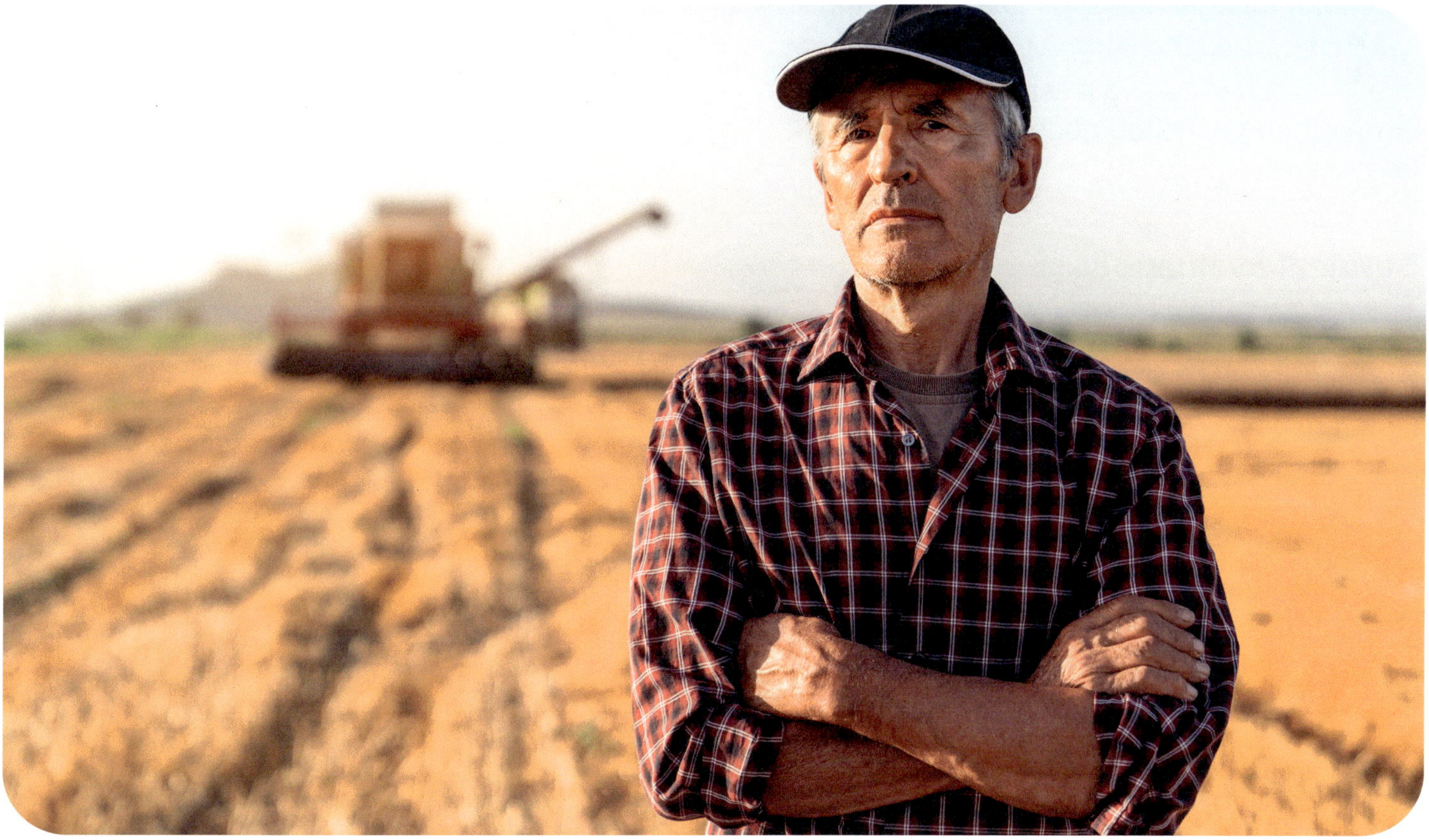

Cutaneous squamous cell carcinoma (cSCC) that has spread to nearby lymph nodes is known as "regional".

First steps

Biopsy

If lymph nodes near the cSCC feel swollen or look abnormal on imaging tests, the next step is a biopsy. The types of biopsies used for squamous cell skin cancer are fine-needle aspiration (FNA) and core needle biopsy. FNA is also known simply as needle biopsy.

Imaging

If biopsy results confirm that the cancer has spread to nearby lymph nodes, a computed tomography (CT) scan of lymph nodes near the cSCC is recommended. The goal is to learn about the number, location, and size of the lymph nodes with cancer. More imaging tests may be needed to see if cancer has spread farther than the lymph nodes, or to help plan treatment.

Surgical evaluation

The results of testing will be considered in order to determine if you are a candidate for surgery to remove the cancerous lesion and nearby lymph nodes.

Treatment

Surgery is recommended to treat squamous cell skin cancer that has spread to nearby lymph nodes. Surgery for regional cSCC involves excision (removal) of the cancerous lesion and nearby lymph nodes. Although surgery is preferred, it may not be an option for one or more reasons. In this case, see *If surgery is not an option* on the next page for information.

Head and neck tumors

Lymph nodes may be removed from one or both sides of the neck during surgery for head and neck tumors. The extent of surgery depends on the number, location, and size of the lymph nodes with cancer. After surgery, radiation therapy is often given to decrease the chance of the tumor returning.

Systemic therapy is sometimes used in addition to radiation therapy after surgery. This may be the case if:

- Lymph nodes with cancer were not removed during surgery, or
- Cancer was found to have grown through the protective outer layer of any lymph nodes removed during surgery (extracapsular or extranodal extension)

In either of these situations, a discussion between different cancer doctors is recommended. If systemic therapy is planned, platinum-based chemotherapy is a recommended option for use with radiation if you can have it. Enrolling in a clinical trial for systemic therapy is also an option. A clinical trial could involve treatment with chemotherapy, targeted therapy, or immunotherapy.

Tumors on other areas of the body

Surgery is also the best way to treat tumors that have spread to other areas of the body if possible. Surgery removes the tumor and nearby lymph nodes. Radiation therapy may be given after surgery to kill leftover cancer cells, especially if there was more than 1 lymph node with cancer or if cancer was found to have grown through the protective outer layer of any lymph nodes removed during surgery.

If surgery is not an option

If you cannot have surgery, a discussion between different cancer physicians to consider your treatment options is recommended. If you can have it, radiation therapy with or without systemic therapy is recommended. Platinum-based chemotherapy is a recommended option for use with radiation.

If radiation therapy is not expected to kill the cancer completely or may damage critical healthy organs, systemic therapy alone is recommended. If you are eligible, immunotherapy with an immune checkpoint inhibitor is a recommended option. Enrolling in a clinical trial for systemic therapy is also an option. A clinical trial could involve treatment with chemotherapy, targeted therapy, or immunotherapy.

If you are not eligible for an immune checkpoint inhibitor or a clinical trial, options for systemic therapy include platinum-based chemotherapy and targeted therapy.

➲ See *When treatment is over* on page 29 for information on monitoring and follow-up care.

Metastatic squamous cell skin cancer

Cancer cells can spread through blood and lymph to form tumors in other areas of the body. This is called metastasis. Squamous cell skin cancer does not metastasize often. For this reason, there is not much research on the best way to treat metastatic squamous cell skin cancer. A discussion between different cancer physicians is recommended to consider your treatment options.

If surgery and/or radiation therapy cannot cure metastatic cSCC, systemic therapy is recommended. If you are eligible, immunotherapy with an immune checkpoint inhibitor is a recommended option. Enrolling in a clinical trial for systemic therapy is another option. A clinical trial could involve treatment with chemotherapy, targeted therapy, or immunotherapy.

If you are not eligible for an immune checkpoint inhibitor or a clinical trial, options for systemic therapy include platinum-based chemotherapy and targeted therapy.

Help for symptoms

Radiation therapy and/or surgery may be used to treat distant tumors that are causing pain or other bothersome side effects. Stereotactic body radiotherapy (SBRT) is a special radiation technique that may be used in some cases. It uses high doses of radiation to small areas to kill cancer cells, and is typically given over 3 to 5 treatments.

Review

- Squamous cell skin cancer that has spread to nearby lymph nodes is called "regional".
- The best way to treat regional cSCC is with surgery to remove the tumor and nearby lymph nodes.
- Radiation therapy with or without systemic therapy is often given after surgery to kill leftover cancer cells.
- If surgery is not possible or not recommended, radiation therapy, systemic therapy, or both may be options.
- If radiation therapy is not expected to kill the cancer completely or may harm critical healthy organs, systemic therapy alone is recommended.
- Although it is uncommon, squamous cell skin cancer can metastasize. Metastatic cSCC that cannot be cured with surgery and/or radiation is treated with systemic therapy.
- Systemic therapy options for metastatic cSCC include immunotherapy or a systemic therapy given in a clinical trial. If you are not a candidate for either of these, your doctor may recommend platinum-based chemotherapy or targeted therapy.

5
When treatment is over

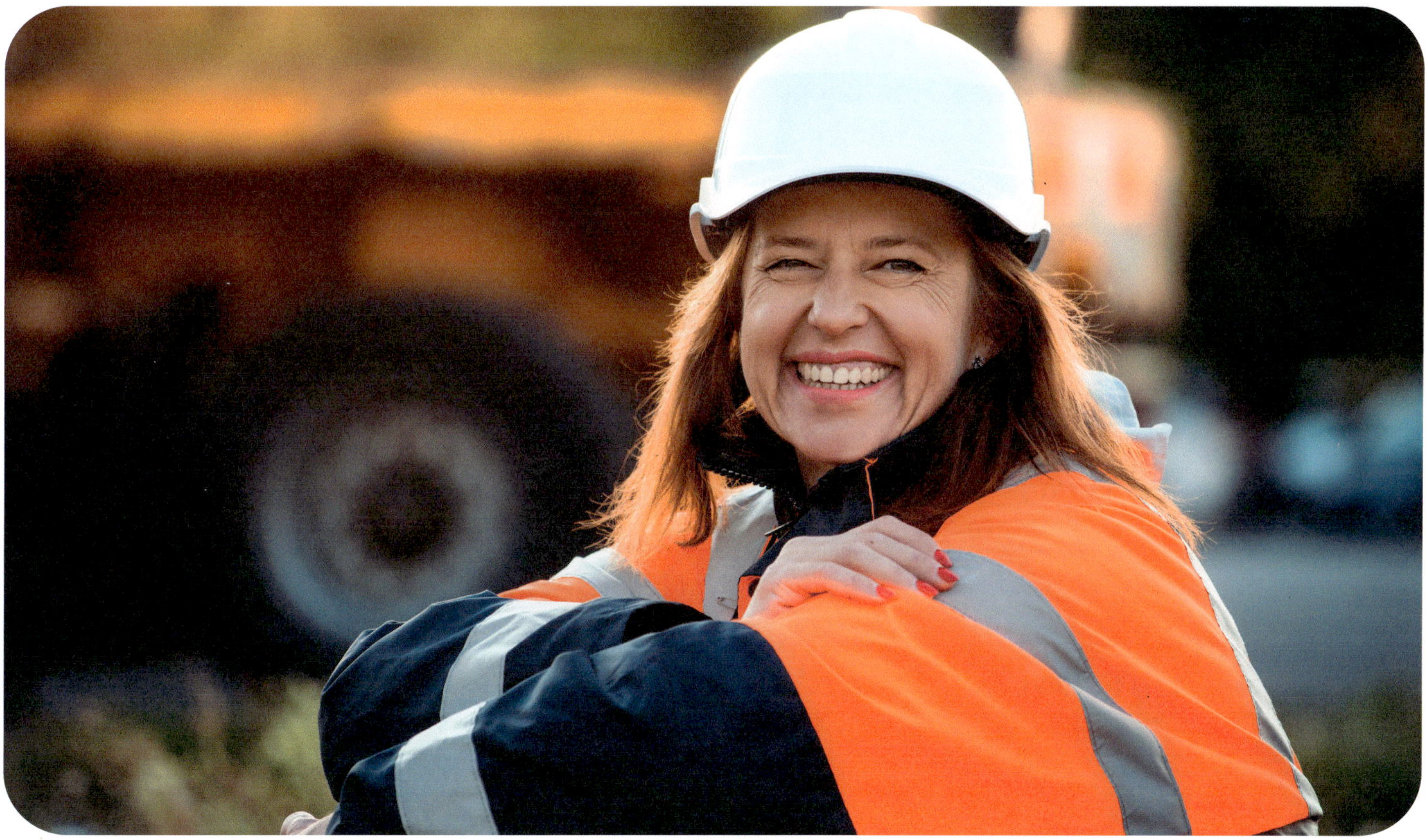

You've finished treatment. Now you may be wondering if—and when—cancer might return. Because you've already had squamous cell skin cancer, you are at higher risk of getting it again. You are also at higher risk of getting other types of skin cancer. This chapter explains how you can help prevent and detect future skin cancers.

Skin exams by your doctor

After finishing treatment, getting regular skin exams to monitor for the return of squamous cell skin cancer is very important. These follow-up exams should include a complete check of the skin on your entire body, as well as the lymph nodes closest to the cancer site. You will be asked to undress and put on a paper gown or drape. Undergarments can be worn during the exam. The gown will be adjusted to allow your doctor to see different areas. How often you should be checked depends on whether the cancer was local (not in nearby lymph nodes) or regional (in nearby lymph nodes).

For local cSCC, monitoring during the first 2 years after treatment is the most important. Exams should occur at least every 3 to 12 months during this time. If no further skin cancer develops in the first 2 years, then exams are spaced out to once or twice a year for another 3 years. After that, having an exam once a year for the rest of your life is recommended by NCCN experts.

For regional cSCC, physical exams with skin checks should be performed every 2 to 3 months for 1 year, every 2 to 4 months for the second year, every 4 to 6 months for another 3 years, and then every 6 to 12 months for life. For patients with regional cSCC, your doctor may want you to have CT scans on a regular basis to look for signs of cancer in nearby lymph nodes or in other parts of your body.

The follow-up exam schedules for both local and regional squamous cell skin cancer are shown in Guide 1.

Guide 1
Follow-up exam schedule

Local cSCC (no spread to lymph nodes)	• First 2 years: Every 3–12 months • Next 3 years: Every 6–12 months • After that: Once every year for life
Regional cSCC (spread to lymph nodes)	• First year: Every 2–3 months • Next year: Every 2–4 months • Next 3 years: Every 4–6 months • After that: Every 6–12 months for life

Steps you can take

Your treatment team should provide you with information about how you can play a role in preventing new skin cancers from forming. The information should cover two important topics—sun protection and skin self-exams.

Sun protection

Protecting your skin from the sun is an important part of preventing future squamous cell carcinomas. One of the best ways to do this is to use a broad-spectrum sunscreen with a sun protection factor (SPF) of 30 or higher. When spending time outside, sunscreen should be reapplied to all exposed areas every 2 hours, or after swimming or sweating. Consider using a face moisturizer with a SPF of 30 or higher on a daily basis.

Physically shielding your skin from the sun with hats and clothing can help protect it. Similar to sun protection factor (SPF) ratings for

Skin exams by your doctor

After finishing treatment, you should have your skin examined by a doctor on a regular basis. How often you should have skin exams depends on whether cancer spread to nearby lymph nodes.

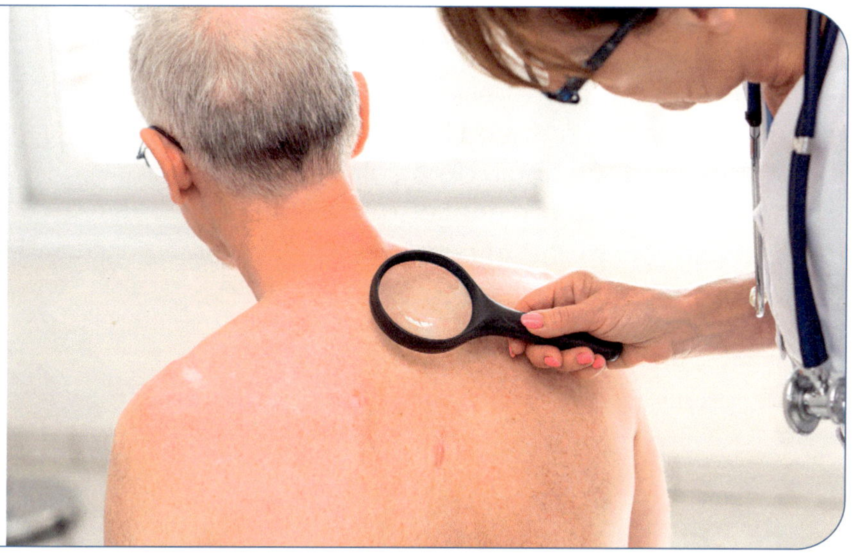

Sun protection

When spending time outside, apply a sunscreen with SPF 30 or higher. Sunscreen should be reapplied to all exposed areas every 2 hours, or after swimming or sweating. Consider using a face moisturizer with SPF of 30 or higher on a daily basis.

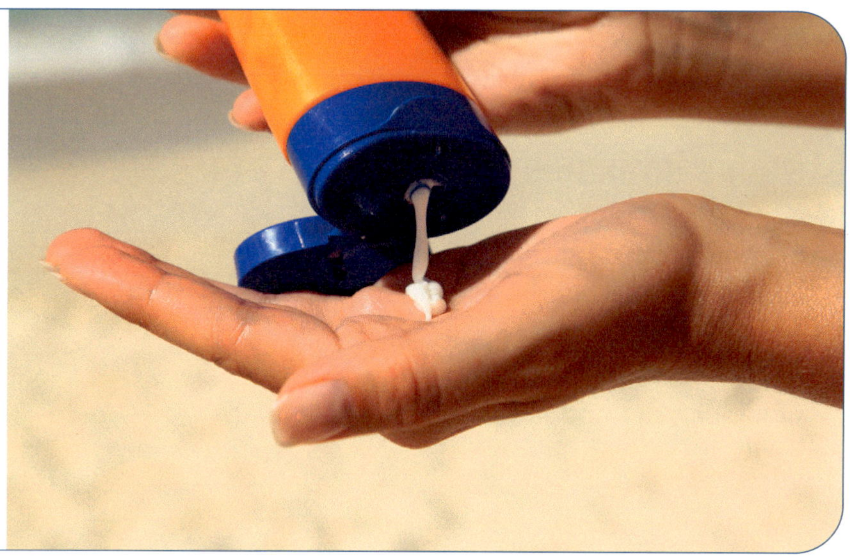

sunscreen, apparel with ultraviolet protection factor (UPF) rating is available. The higher the UPF rating, the better the sun protection. Staying inside (or in the shade) during peak daylight hours is another way to protect your skin. You should never use tanning beds. Your goal is to never get another a sunburn or suntan.

Skin self-exams

Your doctor should also teach you how to examine your skin yourself for signs of cancer. Following the same process each time can make it easier to notice any changes from the last time you checked. A handheld mirror is helpful for seeing hard-to-reach areas. You may also ask a spouse or friend to help you do the exam. Ideally, you should do a self-exam once a month. If you had regional cSCC, meaning that the cancer spread to nearby lymph nodes, your doctor should also teach you how to inspect your lymph nodes for signs of cancer.

Prevention in high-risk patients

Treating squamous cell skin cancer when it first appears can help prevent the cancer from growing into deeper layers of the skin. In people who form cSCCs very easily, however, treatment alone may not be the best strategy. Rather than wait for the cancer to form, there are ways to help prevent squamous cell skin cancer in high-risk individuals. The following groups of people have benefitted in studies where medications were given to help prevent squamous cell skin cancer from forming.

- Organ transplant recipients
- People with xeroderma pigmentosa
- People with psoriasis who have had psoralen and ultraviolet A (PUVA) therapy
- People who have had squamous cell skin cancer more than once
- People with large areas of actinic keratosis

The medicines used to help stop squamous cell skin cancer from forming are described next.

Skin self-exams

In addition to getting full skin exams by your doctor, examining your skin yourself on a regular basis can help spot the return of cancer and find new cancers early.

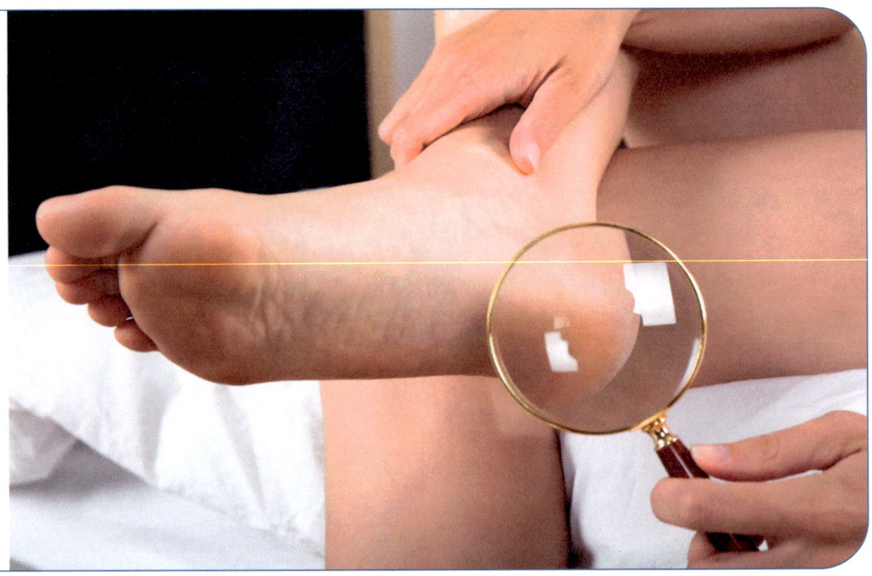

Oral retinoids

When taken by mouth (orally), drugs called retinoids can help prevent squamous cell carcinoma from forming in patients who form actinic keratoses easily. Acitretin (Soriatane®) and isotretinoin are two retinoids used for this purpose.

Oral retinoids can cause drying or chapping of the lips, peeling of the skin, hair disorders, and more extreme side effects. They can also cause birth defects and should therefore be used with extreme caution in women who could become pregnant. People taking these drugs need to have their blood tested on a regular basis.

Oral nicotinamide

Nicotinamide is a form of niacin (vitamin B3). Nicotinamide may help prevent squamous cell carcinoma from returning after treatment and from spreading to distant sites in people at high risk. To prevent squamous cell skin cancer, nicotinamide is taken orally (by mouth) twice a day. No prescription is needed for nicotinamide and it is considered safe.

Widespread sun damage and actinic keratosis

People with widespread actinic keratoses (also known as field cancerization) are at risk of forming multiple cSCCs. See Part 2, *Overview of treatments* for information on superficial therapies including topical treatments and photodynamic therapy. These treatments, especially when repeated every 1–2 years, can reduce the number of cSCCs that form.

Should I be concerned about getting more cSCCs?

Out of 100 people who have had squamous cell skin cancer, about 40 will get a new cSCC within five years—most within the first two years. For this reason, monitoring during the first two years after treatment is very important. NCCN experts recommend having regular skin exams by your doctor, doing skin self-exams, and being strict about sun protection.

Review

- After treatment for cSCC it is important to have your skin examined by your doctor on a regular basis. How often exams are needed depends on whether cancer has spread to nearby lymph nodes.
- Using broad-spectrum sunscreen daily, wearing protective clothing, and staying out of the sun are steps you can take to help prevent new skin cancers from forming.
- In addition to skin checks by your doctor, patients should examine their skin themselves for signs of skin cancer on a regular basis. Patients with regional cSCC should also examine their lymph nodes.
- People at high risk of getting squamous cell skin cancer may benefit from medicines or topical treatments that can help prevent skin cancers from forming.

6 Making treatment decisions

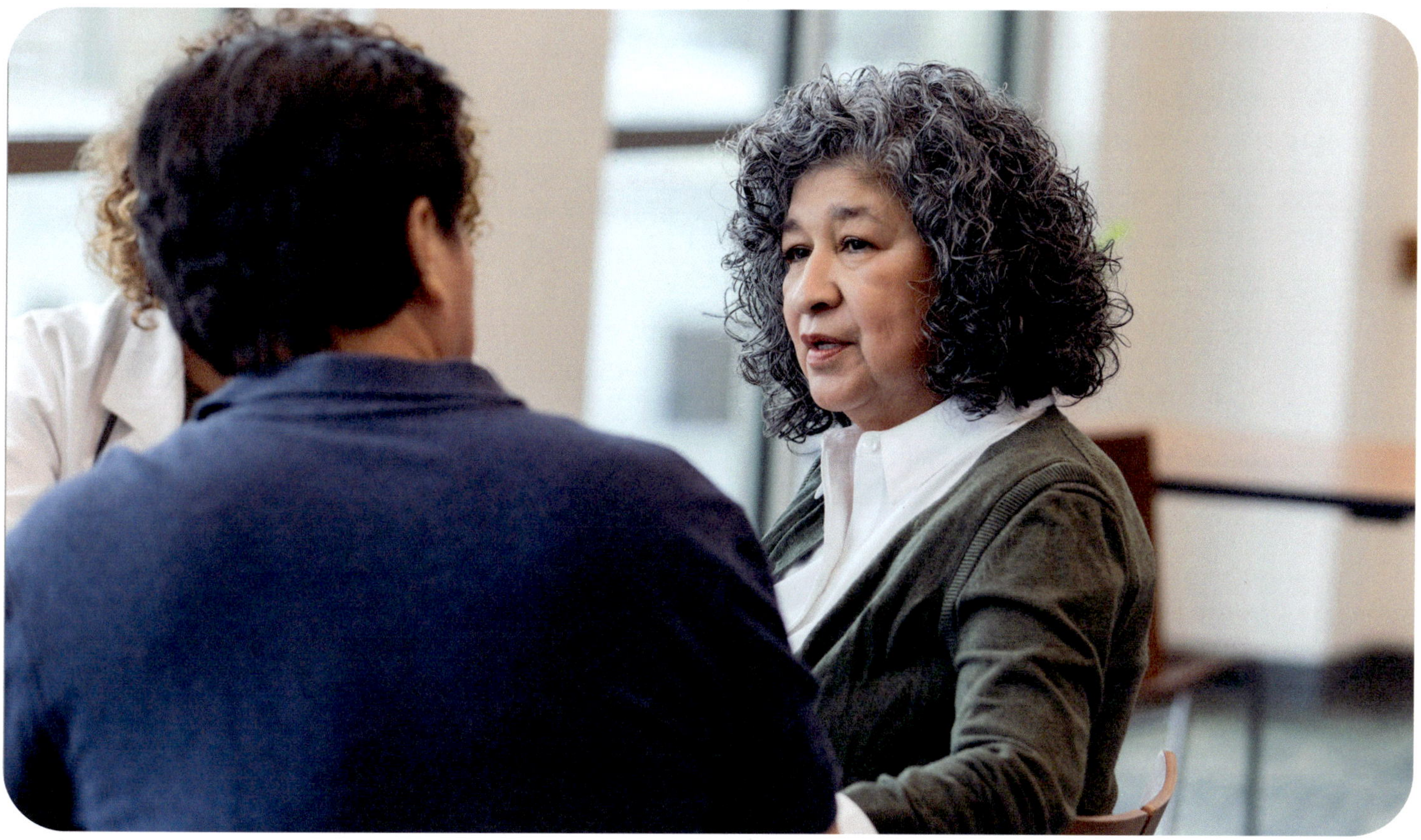

It is important to be comfortable with the cancer treatment you choose. This choice starts with having an open and honest conversation with your doctor.

It's your choice

In shared decision making, you and your doctors share information, discuss the options, and agree on a treatment plan. It starts with an open and honest conversation between you and your doctor.

Treatment decisions are very personal. What is important to you may not be important to someone else. Some things that may play a role in your decision making:

- What you want and how that might differ from what others want
- Your religious and spiritual beliefs
- Your feelings about certain treatments like surgery or chemotherapy
- Your feelings about pain or side effects such as nausea and vomiting
- Cost of treatment, travel to treatment centers, and time away from work
- Quality of life and length of life
- How active you are and the activities that are important to you

Think about what you want from treatment. Discuss openly the risks and benefits of specific treatments and procedures. Weigh options and share concerns with your doctor. If you take the time to build a relationship with your doctor, it will help you feel supported when considering options and making treatment decisions.

Second opinion

It is normal to want to start treatment as soon as possible. While cancer should not be ignored, there is time to have another doctor review your test results and suggest a treatment plan. This is called getting a second opinion, and it is a normal part of cancer care. Even doctors get second opinions!

Things you can do to prepare:

- Check with your insurance company about its rules on second opinions. There may be out-of-pocket costs to see doctors who are not part of your insurance plan.
- Make plans to have copies of all your records sent to the doctor you will see for your second opinion.

Support groups

Many people diagnosed with cancer find support groups to be helpful. Support groups often include people at different stages of treatment. Some people may be newly diagnosed, while others may be finished with treatment. If your hospital or community does not have support groups for people with cancer, check out the websites listed in this book.

Questions to ask your doctors

Possible questions to ask your doctors are listed on the following pages. Feel free to use these questions or come up with your own. Be clear about your goals for treatment and find out what to expect from treatment.

Questions to ask your doctors about testing and results

1. Can you tell me about the symptoms of squamous cell skin cancer?
2. What tests will I have for squamous cell skin cancer?
3. Where and when will the tests take place?
4. How long will the tests take?
5. What are the risks of the tests?
6. How do I prepare for testing?
7. How soon will I know the results, and who will explain them to me?
8. Have any cancer cells spread to other parts of my body?

Questions to ask your doctors about treatment options

1. What are my treatment options?
2. Does this hospital or center offer the best treatment for me?
3. Can you provide me with the research that supports this treatment plan?
4. How often will I get treatment, and will I need more than one treatment?
5. How much time do I have to think about my options?
6. Do I have time to get a second opinion?
7. Am I eligible for surgery?
8. If I undergo surgery, how long will I be in the hospital afterwards?
9. If I undergo surgery, how soon can I return to my normal activities afterwards?

Questions to ask your doctors about side effects

1. What are the side effects of surgery?
2. What are the side effects of radiation therapy?
3. What are the side effects of systemic therapy?
4. When can the side effects start? How long will they last?
5. When should I contact the care team about my side effects?
6. Are there any medications that can prevent or relieve these side effects?
7. Are there any long-term effects of treatment for squamous cell skin cancer?

Questions to ask your doctors about clinical trials

1. Is a clinical trial recommended for me? If so, is there an open trial I can join?
2. Do I have to pay anything to join a clinical trial?
3. How many people will be in the clinical trial?
4. How long does a clinical trial last?
5. How often will I have to go to a hospital or treatment center?
6. Will I be able to get other treatment if this treatment does not work?
7. How will you know if the treatment is working?

Websites

American Cancer Society
cancer.org/cancer/basal-and-squamous-cell-skin-cancer.html

American Academy of Dermatology
aad.org/public/diseases/skin-cancer/squamous-cell-carcinoma

National Cancer Institute (NCI)
cancer.gov/types/skin

Save Your Skin Foundation
saveyourskin.ca/

Skin Cancer Education & Research Foundation
skincancerinfo.org/

Skin Cancer Foundation
skincancer.org

U.S. National Library of Medicine Clinical Trials Database
clinicaltrials.gov

Words to know

actinic keratosis
An area of scaly skin that may become squamous cell skin cancer, but this change is uncommon. Also called solar keratosis.

basal cell carcinoma
The most common type of skin cancer. Also called basal cell skin cancer.

biopsy
A procedure that removes fluid or tissue samples to be tested for a disease.

brachytherapy
A type of radiation therapy used to treat superficial skin cancers that places the radioactive source in close proximity to the tumor.

Bowen's disease
A very early form of squamous cell skin cancer marked by scaly or thickened patches on the skin. Also called squamous cell carcinoma in situ.

clinical trial
A type of research that assesses how well health tests or treatments work in people.

computed tomography (CT)
A test that uses x-rays from many angles to make a picture of the insides of the body.

curettage and electrodesiccation (C&E)
A procedure used to treat skin cancer by scraping away cancerous tissue and destroying remaining cancer cells with an electric needle.

dermis
The second layer of skin that is beneath the outer layer. Contains hair follicles, nerves, sweat glands, oil glands, and blood vessels.

epidermis
The top layer of skin, where squamous cells and basal cells are found.

external beam radiation therapy (EBRT)
A cancer treatment with radiation delivered from a machine outside the body.

subcutaneous tissue
The layer of skin below the dermis that is known for its many fat cells. Also called hypodermis.

immunotherapy
A cancer treatment that stimulates the activity of your body's immune system. By doing so, it improves your body's ability to find and destroy cancer cells.

local therapy
A treatment that is given to a confined area.

Marjolin's ulcer
Squamous cell skin cancer that forms in an area of wounded, inflamed, or scarred skin.

Mohs surgery
A surgical procedure used to treat skin cancer. Layers of cancer-containing tissue are removed and examined under a microscope one at a time until all cancer tissue has been removed. Also called Mohs micrographic surgery.

photodynamic therapy (PDT)
Treatment with drugs that may kill cancer cells when exposed to light.

primary treatment
The main treatment used to rid the body of cancer.

radiation therapy
A treatment that uses intense energy to kill cancer cells. Also called radiotherapy.

squamous cell skin cancer
The second most common type of skin cancer. Most often caused by many years of sun

exposure or multiple sunburns. Also called cutaneous squamous cell carcinoma (cSCC).

SCC in situ
A very early form of squamous cell skin cancer marked by scaly or thickened patches on the skin. Also called Bowen's disease.

sun protection factor (SPF)
A rating of protection against ultraviolet rays.

surgical margin
The normal-looking ring of tissue around a tumor that is removed during surgery.

systemic therapy
A type of treatment that works throughout the body.

targeted therapy
A cancer treatment that may target and attack specific types of cancer cells.

NCCN Contributors

This patient guide is based on the NCCN Clinical Practice Guidelines in Oncology (NCCN Guidelines®) for Squamous Cell Skin Cancer. It was adapted, reviewed, and published with help from the following people:

Dorothy A. Shead, MS
Director, Patient Information Operations

Laura J. Hanisch, PsyD
Medical Writer/Patient Information Specialist

Erin Vidic, MA
Medical Writer

Rachael Clarke
Senior Medical Copyeditor

Tanya Fischer, MEd, MSLIS
Medical Writer

Kim Williams
Creative Services Manager

Susan Kidney
Graphic Design Specialist

The NCCN Guidelines® for Squamous Cell Skin Cancer, Version 2.2020 were developed by the following NCCN Panel Members:

Chrysalyne D. Schmults, MD/Chair
Dana-Farber/Brigham and Women's Cancer Center

Rachel Blitzblau, MD, PhD/Vice Chair
Duke Cancer Institute

Sumaira Z. Aasi, MD
Stanford Cancer Institute

Murad Alam, MD
Robert H. Lurie Comprehensive Cancer Center of Northwestern University

James S. Andersen, MD
City of Hope National Medical Center

Jeremy Bordeaux, MD, MPH
Case Comprehensive Cancer Center/ University Hospitals Seidman Cancer Center and Cleveland Clinic Taussig Cancer Institute

Glen M. Bowen, MD
Huntsman Cancer Institute at the University of Utah

William Carson III, MD
The Ohio State University Comprehensive Cancer Center - James Cancer Hospital and Solove Research Institute

Pei-Ling Chen, MD, PhD
Moffitt Cancer Center

Carlo M. Contreras, MD
O'Neal Comprehensive Cancer Center at UAB

Mackenzie Daly, MD
Siteman Cancer Center at Barnes-Jewish Hospital and Washington University School of Medicine

Gregory A. Daniels, MD, PhD
UC San Diego Moores Cancer Center

Dominick DiMaio, MD
Fred & Pamela Buffett Cancer Center

*Jeffrey M. Farma, MD
Fox Chase Cancer Center

Kristopher Fisher, MD
St. Jude Children's Research Hospital/ University of Tennessee Health Science Center

Karthik Ghosh, MD
Mayo Clinic Cancer Center

Roy C. Grekin, MD
UCSF Helen Diller Family Comprehensive Cancer Center

Kelly Harms, MD, PhD
University of Michigan Rogel Cancer Center

Alan L. Ho, MD, PhD
Memorial Sloan Kettering Cancer Center

Donald Lawrence, MD
Massachusetts General Hospital Cancer Center

Karl D. Lewis, MD
University of Colorado Cancer Center

*Manisha Loss, MD
Sidney Kimmel Comprehensive Cancer Center at Johns Hopkins

*John Nicholas Lukens, MD
Abramson Cancer Center at the University of Pennsylvania

Kishwer S. Nehal, MD
Memorial Sloan Kettering Cancer Center

Paul Nghiem, MD, PhD
Fred Hutchinson Cancer Research Center/ Seattle Cancer Care Alliance

Igor Puzanov, MD, MSCI, FACP
Roswell Park Cancer Institute

Aleksandar Sekulic, MD, PhD
Mayo Clinic Cancer Center

Ashok R. Shaha, MD
Memorial Sloan Kettering Cancer Center

William Stebbins, MD
Vanderbilt-Ingram Cancer Center

Valencia Thomas, MD
The University of Texas MD Anderson Cancer Center

Yaohui G. Xu, MD, PhD
University of Wisconsin Carbone Cancer Center

NCCN Staff

Anita Engh, PhD
Oncology Scientist/Medical Writer

Mary Dwyer, MS
Director, Guidelines Operations

* Reviewed this patient guide. For disclosures, visit NCCN.org/about/disclosure.aspx.

NCCN Cancer Centers

Abramson Cancer Center
at the University of Pennsylvania
Philadelphia, Pennsylvania
800.789.7366 • pennmedicine.org/cancer

Fred & Pamela Buffett Cancer Center
Omaha, Nebraska
402.559.5600 • unmc.edu/cancercenter

Case Comprehensive Cancer Center/
University Hospitals Seidman Cancer
Center and Cleveland Clinic Taussig
Cancer Institute
Cleveland, Ohio
800.641.2422 • UH Seidman Cancer Center
uhhospitals.org/services/cancer-services
866.223.8100 • CC Taussig Cancer Institute
my.clevelandclinic.org/departments/cancer
216.844.8797 • Case CCC
case.edu/cancer

City of Hope National Medical Center
Los Angeles, California
800.826.4673 • cityofhope.org

Dana-Farber/Brigham and
Women's Cancer Center
Boston, Massachusetts
617.732.5500
youhaveus.org

Massachusetts General Hospital
Cancer Center
617.726.5130
massgeneral.org/cancer-center

Duke Cancer Institute
Durham, North Carolina
888.275.3853 • dukecancerinstitute.org

Fox Chase Cancer Center
Philadelphia, Pennsylvania
888.369.2427 • foxchase.org

Huntsman Cancer Institute
at the University of Utah
Salt Lake City, Utah
800.824.2073
huntsmancancer.org

Fred Hutchinson Cancer
Research Center/Seattle
Cancer Care Alliance
Seattle, Washington
206.606.7222 • seattlecca.org
206.667.5000 • fredhutch.org

The Sidney Kimmel Comprehensive
Cancer Center at Johns Hopkins
Baltimore, Maryland
410.955.8964
www.hopkinskimmelcancercenter.org

Robert H. Lurie Comprehensive
Cancer Center of Northwestern
University
Chicago, Illinois
866.587.4322 • cancer.northwestern.edu

Mayo Clinic Cancer Center
Phoenix/Scottsdale, Arizona
Jacksonville, Florida
Rochester, Minnesota
480.301.8000 • Arizona
904.953.0853 • Florida
507.538.3270 • Minnesota
mayoclinic.org/cancercenter

Memorial Sloan Kettering
Cancer Center
New York, New York
800.525.2225 • mskcc.org

Moffitt Cancer Center
Tampa, Florida
888.663.3488 • moffitt.org

The Ohio State University
Comprehensive Cancer Center -
James Cancer Hospital and
Solove Research Institute
Columbus, Ohio
800.293.5066 • cancer.osu.edu

O'Neal Comprehensive
Cancer Center at UAB
Birmingham, Alabama
800.822.0933 • uab.edu/onealcancercenter

Roswell Park Comprehensive
Cancer Center
Buffalo, New York
877.275.7724 • roswellpark.org

Siteman Cancer Center at Barnes-
Jewish Hospital and Washington
University School of Medicine
St. Louis, Missouri
800.600.3606 • siteman.wustl.edu

St. Jude Children's Research Hospital
The University of Tennessee
Health Science Center
Memphis, Tennessee
866.278.5833 • stjude.org
901.448.5500 • uthsc.edu

Stanford Cancer Institute
Stanford, California
877.668.7535 • cancer.stanford.edu

UC San Diego Moores Cancer Center
La Jolla, California
858.822.6100• cancer.ucsd.edu

UCLA Jonsson
Comprehensive Cancer Center
Los Angeles, California
310.825.5268 • cancer.ucla.edu

UCSF Helen Diller Family
Comprehensive Cancer Center
San Francisco, California
800.689.8273 • cancer.ucsf.edu

University of Colorado Cancer Center
Aurora, Colorado
720.848.0300 • coloradocancercenter.org

University of Michigan
Rogel Cancer Center
Ann Arbor, Michigan
800.865.1125 • rogelcancercenter.org

The University of Texas
MD Anderson Cancer Center
Houston, Texas
844.269.5922 • mdanderson.org

University of Wisconsin
Carbone Cancer Center
Madison, Wisconsin
608.265.1700 • uwhealth.org/cancer

UT Southwestern Simmons
Comprehensive Cancer Center
Dallas, Texas
214.648.3111 • utsouthwestern.edu/simmons

Vanderbilt-Ingram Cancer Center
Nashville, Tennessee
877.936.8422 • vicc.org

Yale Cancer Center/
Smilow Cancer Hospital
New Haven, Connecticut
855.4.SMILOW • yalecancercenter.org

Notes

Index

Made in the USA
Monee, IL
12 September 2026

62974523R00031